ATKINS DIET COOKBOOK FOR EPILEPSY (2024-2025)

Seizure-Free Living: Discover Delicious, Low-Carb Recipes to Effectively Manage Epilepsy Symptoms with the Proven Atkins Diet

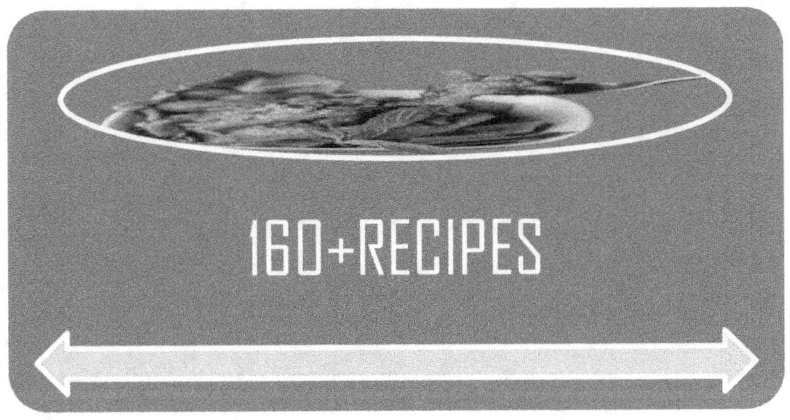

DR.D.JOHNSTON

CONTENTS

INTRODUCTION

MARK STORY TO WELLNESS

Dr. D. Johnston, Mark's childhood friend and now a famous nutritionist, still chuckles when recalling Mark's early culinary attempts. "Burnt toast was a gourmet meal in our college days," he says with a warm smile. "Mark's idea of sustenance involved ramen noodles and questionable frozen dinners." Little did anyone know that the man who once fought to boil water would blossom into a wellness guru, crafting delicious and nutritious recipes that inspire countless others.

The turning point came during a particularly stressful time in Mark's life. Juggling a demanding job, a new marriage, and the yearning for a healthier lifestyle, Mark found himself constantly depleted. Fast food became a crutch, and his energy levels dropped. Witnessing his friend's struggle, Dr. Johnston chose to intervene.

"We started small," Dr. Johnston remembers. "Simple swaps like replacing sugary drinks with water and incorporating more fruits and veggies into his diet. We explored the local farmer's market together, and Mark was amazed by the bright colors and fresh flavors."

A spark sparked within Mark. He began devouring cookbooks, experimenting with ingredients, and slowly but surely, the kitchen changed from a battleground to a playground. "There were failures, of course," Dr. Johnston laughs. "Smoke alarms went off, and a few questionable foods ended up straight in the compost bin. But Mark never gave up. He saw cooking as a journey of discovery, and each mistake was an important learning experience."

As Mark's culinary skills blossomed, so did his general well-being. He had more energy, his focus sharpened, and a fresh sense of calm pervaded his life. "Food wasn't just sustenance anymore," Dr. Johnston says. "It became a powerful tool for change. Mark realized that nourishing his body with the right ingredients had a profound effect on his mind, mood, and overall health."

Witnessing Mark's transformation, Dr. Johnston urged him to share his newfound passion with the world. "Mark's enthusiasm is infectious," he says. "He has a way of making healthy eating seem easy, exciting even. This cookbook is a culmination of his journey, an ode to the power of food to heal and inspire."

Dr. Johnston thinks Mark's story resonates because it's real. "It's not about achieving some unattainable ideal," he explains. "It's about growth, not perfection. Mark's journey is an inspiration to anyone who wants to feel better, live healthier, and rediscover the joy of cooking." So, with a twinkle in his eye, Dr. Johnston continues, "Who knew the boy who once burnt toast would become a culinary alchemist, transforming not just his own life, but the lives of countless others through the magic of food and wellness?"

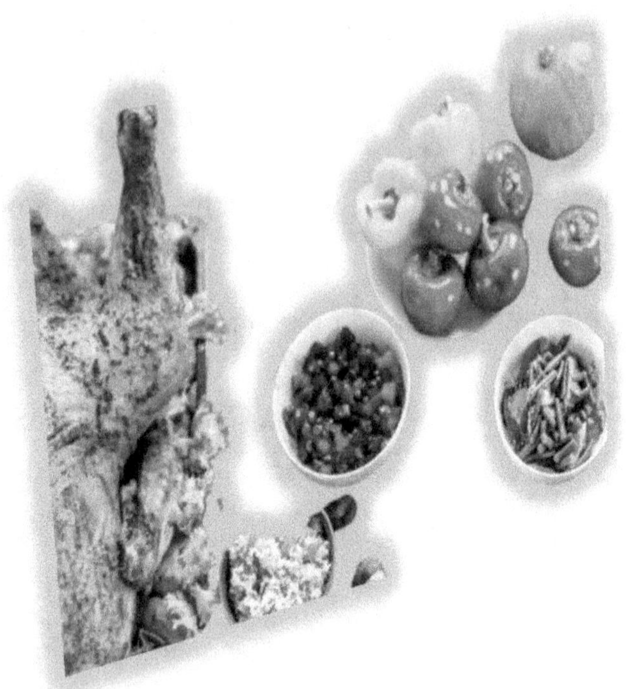

Chapter 1:

Foreword

A Note from the Author

Thanks for coming to the Atkins Diet Cookbook for Epilepsy. I'm excited to share this resource with you because I'm a doctor and have seen directly how dietary changes can change people's lives. The ketogenic ideas behind the Atkins Diet have shown a lot of promise in helping people with seizures, especially when other treatments don't work. This cookbook is meant to be a useful resource. It includes not only tasty meals but also the information you need to start and stick to this diet plan.

Thanks for reading this book. I hope it helps you get healthier and better handle your seizures. Each recipe has been created with care, balancing nutritional needs with flavors that delight the palate. I truly hope that these meals bring you happiness and good health.

Many thanks,

Dr. D. Johnston

Thank you notes

This cookbook would not have been possible without the help and encouragement of many individuals.

First, I want to thank the patients and their families for giving me ideas for this work. Your resilience and drive are truly remarkable.

I am truly grateful to my colleagues and the medical community for their ongoing study and commitment to understanding epilepsy and dietary therapies. Your thoughts and dedication have been invaluable.

A special thank you to my family and friends for their unwavering support and patience throughout the making of this book. Your trust in my work has been a constant source of motivation.

Lastly, I would like to recognize the pioneers of the Atkins Diet and ketogenic research. Your groundbreaking work has paved the way for innovative treatment choices that improve the lives of many.

Thank you all for your donations and support.

Sincerely,

Dr. D. Johnston

Chapter 2:

Understanding the Atkins Diet

History and Principles of the Atkins Diet

The Atkins Diet, a low-carbohydrate eating plan, was first promoted by Dr. Robert C. Atkins in the early 1970s. Dr. Atkins, a cardiologist, developed the diet after extensive study on the effects of carbohydrates on body weight and health. His findings were published in the book "Dr. Atkins' Diet Revolution," which quickly gained popularity due to its novel approach to weight loss and its promise of significant results without the hunger usually associated with dieting.

History

Dr. Atkins' journey began in the 1960s when he came across a study paper discussing the benefits of a low-carbohydrate diet. Intrigued by the findings, he chose to test the approach on himself and some of his patients. The results were striking: major weight loss and improvements in several health markers.

Encouraged by these outcomes, Dr. Atkins began to advocate for a low-carb lifestyle, stressing its potential to fight obesity and related health issues.

The diet's popularity surged in the 1990s and early 2000s, leading to the release of several more books by Dr. Atkins and a series of updates to his original plan. Despite facing criticism from some in the medical community, the Atkins Diet kept a strong following due to its effectiveness and the growing body of research supporting low-carb eating.

Principles

The Atkins Diet is based on the concept that reducing carbohydrate intake forces the body to burn fat for fuel, leading to weight loss and better health. The key concepts of the Atkins Diet include:

- **Carbohydrate Restriction:** The diet limits carbohydrate intake, especially refined carbs and sugars, to encourage the body to enter a state of ketosis, where it burns fat for energy.

- **Protein and Fat Emphasis**: It promotes the consumption of proteins and healthy fats, which are more satiating than carbohydrates and help keep muscle mass while losing weight.

- **Gradual Reintroduction of Carbs:** The diet includes phases that gradually reintroduce carbohydrates, helping people find their ideal carb balance for weight maintenance.

- **Focus on Whole Foods:** The diet supports the consumption of whole, unprocessed foods, such as vegetables, meats, fish, and healthy fats, while avoiding processed foods and sugars.

Phases of the Atkins Diet

The Atkins Diet is structured into four phases, each with specific goals and rules to help people transition from weight loss to weight maintenance.

Phase 1: Induction

The Induction phase is the most restrictive phase, meant to kickstart weight loss by putting the body into ketosis. Key guidelines for this time include:

- Carbohydrate Limit: Intake is restricted to 20 grams of net carbs per day, mainly from leafy greens and non-starchy vegetables.

- Protein and Fat: High amount of proteins and healthy fats from meats, fish, eggs, and oils.

- Avoidance of Certain Foods: No fruits, bread, pasta, grains, starchy veggies, or dairy products other than cheese, cream, and butter.

- Duration: This phase lasts for at least two weeks but can be extended for those with major weight loss goals.

Phase 2: Balancing

The Balancing phase allows for a gradual increase in carbohydrate diet while continuing weight loss. Key rules include:

- Raised Carbs: Daily net carb intake is raised by 5 grams per week, focusing on nutrient-dense and low-glycemic foods like nuts, seeds, and berries.

- Monitoring Tolerance: Individuals watch their body's response to added carbs to find their personal carbohydrate tolerance level for continued weight loss.

- Continued Restrictions: Still avoid sugary sugars, white flour, and high-carb foods.

- Duration: This phase continues until the person is within 10 pounds of their goal weight.

Phase 3: Pre-Maintenance

The Pre-control phase prepares the body for long-term weight control by further increasing carbohydrate intake. Key rules include:

- Gradual Increase: Daily net carb intake is increased by 10 grams per week, adding a wider range of foods such as legumes, whole grains, and more fruits.
- Identifying Tolerance: Individuals find their critical carbohydrate level for maintenance (CCLM), which is the highest number of carbs they can eat without gaining weight.
- Fine-Tuning: This phase includes fine-tuning the diet to maintain weight loss and prevent weight regain.
- Duration: This phase lasts until the person has maintained their goal weight for at least a month.

Phase 4: Lifetime Maintenance

The Lifetime Maintenance phase is meant for long-term adherence, ensuring that individuals can keep their weight loss and health improvements indefinitely. Key rules include:

- Sustainable Eating: Continue to eat a balanced meal with controlled carbohydrate intake based on the individual's CCLM.
- Flexibility: Allow occasional indulgences while avoiding a return to high-carb eating habits.
- Monitoring: Regularly check weight and health markers to make adjustments as needed.
- Lifelong Commitment: This phase emphasizes the importance of maintaining the dietary changes for life to sustain the benefits gained.

Benefits of Low-Carb Eating

Low-carb meals, such as the Atkins Diet, offer a range of benefits beyond weight loss. These benefits are supported by a growing body of scientific study.

Weight Loss and Maintenance

One of the major benefits of low-carb eating is its effectiveness for weight loss and maintenance. By reducing carbohydrate intake, the body is pushed to burn fat for fuel, leading to significant weight loss. Studies have shown that low-carb diets can be more effective than low-fat diets for long-term weight loss and maintenance, partly due to their ability to reduce hunger and improve satiety.

Improved Blood Sugar Control

Low-carb diets are particularly beneficial for people with diabetes or insulin resistance. By reducing carbohydrate intake, these diets help stabilize blood sugar levels and improve insulin sensitivity. Many individuals on low-carb diets find reduced need for medication and better overall blood sugar control.

Enhanced Heart Health

Contrary to earlier concerns about the impact of high-fat diets on heart health, recent research suggests that low-carb diets can improve several cardiovascular risk factors. These include decreases in triglycerides, increases in HDL (good) cholesterol, and improvements in blood pressure. Some studies show that low-carb diets can also reduce inflammation and improve arterial function.

Increased Energy and Mental Clarity

Many people report increased energy levels and better mental clarity on a low-carb diet. By providing a steady supply of energy from fats and ketones, low-carb diets can avoid the energy crashes associated with high-carb eating patterns. Additionally, ketones are a more efficient fuel source for the brain, which may explain the enhanced cognitive function described by many low-carb dieters.

Reduced Risk of Chronic Diseases

Low-carb diets have been linked to a reduced chance of several chronic diseases, including type 2 diabetes, metabolic syndrome, and certain cancers. By improving metabolic health, reducing inflammation, and stabilizing blood sugar levels, low-carb eating can add to long-term health and disease prevention.

Better Digestive Health

Low-carb diets stress whole, unprocessed foods, which can improve digestive health. Many individuals experience relief from stomach issues such as bloating, gas, and indigestion when they eliminate processed foods and high-carb items from their diet. The focus on vegetables and healthy fats also supports a healthy gut microbiome.

Chapter 3:
Epilepsy and Diet

Overview of Epilepsy

Epilepsy is a neurological disease characterized by recurrent, unprovoked seizures. These seizures are the result of abnormal electrical activity in the brain, which can cause a variety of symptoms based on the part of the brain affected. Epilepsy affects people of all ages, and its severity and effect can vary widely from person to person.

Causes and Risk Factors

The exact cause of epilepsy is often unknown, but several factors can add to its development, including:

- Genetic Factors: Some forms of epilepsy are hereditary, showing a genetic predisposition to the disorder.

- Brain Injuries: Trauma to the brain from accidents, infections, or strokes can lead to seizures.

- Developmental Disorders: Conditions like autism and neurofibromatosis are linked with a higher risk of epilepsy.

- Prenatal Injuries: Injuries or infections during pregnancy can affect brain development and increase the chance of epilepsy in the child.

• Types of Seizures

- Seizures in epilepsy can be generally categorized into two types:

- Focal Seizures: These start in a specific area of the brain and can cause a variety of symptoms, such as unusual feelings, movements, or behaviors.

- Generalized Seizures: These affect both sides of the brain from the onset and can cause loss of consciousness, convulsions, or muscle stiffness.

Diagnosis and Treatment

Diagnosing epilepsy typically includes a combination of medical history, neurological exams, and diagnostic tests such as electroencephalograms (EEGs) and imaging studies (MRI or CT scans). Treatment choices include:

- Medications: Anti-epileptic drugs (AEDs) are the most common treatment and can help control seizures in many people.
- Surgery: In cases where seizures originate from a specific area of the brain that can be safely removed, surgery may be a possibility.
- Therapies: Vagus nerve stimulation (VNS), responsive neurostimulation (RNS), and ketogenic diets are alternative therapies that can help control seizures.
- Lifestyle Changes: Avoiding seizure triggers, getting enough sleep, and managing stress are important parts of managing epilepsy.

The Role of Diet in Managing Epilepsy

Dietary therapy has long been recognized as a valuable method to managing epilepsy, especially in cases where medications are ineffective or cause undesirable side effects. The most well-known dietary treatment is the ketogenic diet, which was developed in the 1920s especially for epilepsy management.

Ketogenic Diet

The ketogenic diet is a high-fat, low-carbohydrate diet that mimics the metabolic state of fasting, causing a state of ketosis. In ketosis, the body burns fat for energy instead of carbohydrates, creating ketones as a byproduct. These ketones have been found to have anticonvulsant effects, reducing the frequency and severity of seizures in many people with epilepsy.

Mechanisms of Action

Several mechanisms have been offered to explain how ketogenic diets help control seizures:

- Ketone Bodies: The production of ketone bodies during ketosis may stabilize neuronal activity and lower seizure frequency.

- Energy Metabolism: By changing the way the brain uses energy, ketogenic diets may help protect against seizures.

- Neurotransmitter Balance: These diets may affect the balance of neurotransmitters, reducing excitatory signals and enhancing inhibitory ones.

- Anti-inflammatory Effects: Ketogenic diets have been shown to lower inflammation, which may play a role in seizure activity.

How the Atkins Diet Helps Epilepsy

The Atkins Diet, while originally created for weight loss, shares many principles with the ketogenic diet and has been adapted for epilepsy management. Its effectiveness in reducing seizure frequency and severity is widely known, especially in individuals who do not respond well to traditional medications.

Inducing Ketosis

Like the ketogenic diet, the Atkins Diet restricts carbohydrate intake, pushing the body to enter a state of ketosis. This metabolic shift is important for producing ketones, which have anticonvulsant properties.

- Low Carbohydrate Intake: The Atkins Diet starts with a very low carbohydrate intake during the Induction phase, usually around 20 grams of net carbs per day, which is sufficient to induce ketosis.

- High Fat and Protein: Emphasis on eating healthy fats and adequate protein helps maintain ketosis while providing necessary nutrients and promoting satiety.

Benefits for Epilepsy Management

The Atkins Diet offers several benefits for treating epilepsy, including:

- Seizure Control: Many individuals with epilepsy experience a major reduction in seizure frequency and severity when following a low-carbohydrate diet. This effect is particularly noticeable in cases of drug-resistant epilepsy.

- Improved Tolerability: Compared to the standard ketogenic diet, the Atkins Diet is often easier to follow and more palatable, improving long-term adherence.

- Nutritional Balance: The Atkins Diet includes a variety of nutrient-dense foods, ensuring that people receive important vitamins and minerals while maintaining ketosis.

Practical Considerations

Implementing the Atkins Diet for epilepsy requires careful planning and monitoring to ensure it is both successful and nutritionally balanced. Key factors include:

- Medical Supervision: It is important to undertake dietary therapy for epilepsy under the guidance of a healthcare professional, especially for children or individuals with other medical conditions.

- Nutrient Monitoring: Regular monitoring of nutrient intake and blood levels is important to avoid deficiencies and ensure overall health.

- Individualization: The diet may need to be tailored to individual needs and preferences, with changes to carbohydrate intake and food choices based on response and tolerability.

Chapter 4:

Getting Started

Kitchen Essentials

Embrace these tools to make your Atkins for Epilepsy journey smooth sailing:

- Sharp Knives and Cutting Boards: Invest in good quality knives for easy chopping and slicing. Choose different cutting boards for meat and vegetables to avoid cross-contamination.

- Mixing Bowls: A range of sizes will come in handy for mixing ingredients, preparing batters, and serving salads.

- Measuring Cups and Spoons: Accuracy is key in following recipes. Get a set of dry and liquid measuring cups and spoons for precise amount control.

- Non-Stick Pans: These are perfect for cooking meat, fish, and eggs with minimal oil, reducing added fat.

- Baking Sheets and Racks: Perfect for roasting veggies, meats, and baking low-carb treats.

- Blender/Food Processor: These tools can be lifesavers for pureeing cauliflower rice, making healthy dips and sauces, and grinding nuts and seeds.

- Spiralizer: This gadget helps create vegetable noodles from zucchini, squash, or sweet potatoes, giving a low-carb pasta alternative.

- Slow Cooker: A lifesaver for busy days. Throw in your items and come home to a delicious, low-carb meal.

- Storage Containers: Invest in airtight containers for storing leftovers, cooked meats, and prepped veggies.

Grocery Shopping Tips

Planning your grocery list is crucial for staying on track with the Atkins for Epilepsy method. Here are some key points:

- Prioritize Protein: Stock your fridge with various protein sources like fatty fish (salmon, tuna), lean foods (chicken breast, ground turkey), and eggs. Consider including some plant-based protein choices like tofu, tempeh, and lentils (in moderation).

- Focus on Low-Carb Veggies: Fill your cart with leafy greens (spinach, kale), broccoli, cauliflower, asparagus, bell peppers, and mushrooms. These provide important nutrients while keeping your carb intake low.

- Healthy Fats are Friends: Opt for healthy fats like olive oil, avocado oil, nuts, and seeds. These provide satiety, fuel your body, and enhance nutrient absorption.

- Limited Fruits: Fruits are higher in carbs. Choose berries like raspberries and strawberries in moderation.

- Minimize Processed Foods and Sugary Drinks: Avoid processed meats, sugary sauces, packed snacks, and sugary drinks. These can cause seizures and derail your dietary efforts.

- Read Food Labels Carefully: Become a label-reading pro. Look for the net carbs (total carbs minus dietary fiber) amount and aim for foods that fall within your personalized carb limit set by your healthcare professional.

Meal Planning and Prep

Planning your meals ahead of time keeps you on track and stops unhealthy temptations. Here's how to make it work:

- Plan Your Week's Meals: Dedicate some time each week to plan your meals. Consider your plan and choose recipes that are quick and easy to prepare on busy days.

- Create a Grocery List: Based on your meal plan, make a detailed grocery list to avoid impulse purchases at the store.

- Prep in Advance: Wash and chop veggies, cook protein sources in bulk, and pre-portion snacks for the week. This saves time during busy moments.

- Cook Once, Eat Twice: Double or triple recipes for extras. This saves cooking time throughout the week.

- Prepare Low-Carb Staples: Pre-cook a batch of cauliflower rice, bake a tray of chicken breasts, or hard-boil a dozen eggs for quick and easy meal adds.

Reading Nutrition Labels for Atkins for Epilepsy

Understanding food labels is key to understanding the Atkins for Epilepsy approach. Here's what to pay close attention to:

- Serving Size: Be aware of serving sizes. The information on the label is based on one serving, and you might be eating more than that.

- Total Carbs: This includes all types of carbs in the food.

- Dietary Fiber: Fiber is not fully digested by the body and doesn't significantly raise blood sugar levels. Subtract dietary fiber from total carbs to get the net carbs amount.

Chapter 5:

Introduction to Induction Phase

Goals and Guidelines for Atkins for Epilepsy

The main goal of the Atkins for Epilepsy approach is to achieve ketosis, a metabolic state where your body burns fat for fuel instead of glucose (derived from carbohydrates). This can possibly lead to a reduction in seizure frequency for some individuals with epilepsy.

Additional possible benefits may include:

Improved brain function

Weight loss (if wanted)

Enhanced happiness and energy levels

Guidelines

The Atkins for Epilepsy follows a similar framework to the normal Atkins diet, but with stricter carbohydrate restrictions. Here's a breakdown of the different phases:

- Induction (Initial Phase): This phase is usually the most restrictive, lasting for 2-4 weeks. It aims to reach ketosis quickly by limiting net carbs to 20-25 grams per day.

- Ongoing Low-Carb Phase (OLC): Once in ketosis, you gradually increase your net carb intake to an amount that maintains ketosis. This level will be set by your healthcare professional based on your individual needs and response to the diet.

- Pre-Maintenance (Optional): This phase (optional for some) allows for occasional higher-carb days to promote metabolic flexibility and possibly prevent plateaus in weight loss (if applicable).

- **Important Considerations:**

- Individualization: The Atkins for Epilepsy needs to be adjusted. A healthcare professional will set your specific carb limit and monitor your progress throughout the process.

- Electrolyte Balance: The Atkins diet can cause electrolyte abnormalities. Ensure adequate intake of sodium, potassium, and magnesium through diet or supplements under your doctor's direction.

- Hydration: Staying well-hydrated is important. Drink plenty of water throughout the day.

- Blood Ketone Monitoring: Your doctor may suggest monitoring your blood ketone levels to confirm ketosis and adjust your carb intake accordingly.

Foods to Eat and Avoid on Atkins for Epilepsy

Foods to Emphasize:

- Protein Sources: Fatty fish (salmon, tuna), lean foods (chicken breast, ground turkey), eggs, tofu, tempeh (in moderation).

- Low-Carb Vegetables: Leafy greens (spinach, kale), broccoli, cauliflower, asparagus, bell peppers, mushrooms, zucchini, eggplant.

- Healthy Fats: Olive oil, avocado oil, nuts (almonds, walnuts, macadamias), seeds (chia, flax), MCT oil (check your doctor first).

- Limited Fruits: Berries (raspberries, strawberries) in moderation.

- Low-Carb Dairy (Optional): Unsweetened full-fat yogurt, cheese (hard cheeses like cheddar).

Foods to Avoid or Limit:

- Grains and Starches: Bread, pasta, rice, cereals, crackers, starchy veggies (corn, potatoes, peas).

- Sugary Drinks: Soda, juice, sweetened coffee, sports drinks.

- Sugary Fruits: Most fruits except berries.

- Legumes (Limited): Beans, beans (due to higher carb content).

- Processed Foods: Packaged snacks, sugary sauces, processed meats (lunch meats, hot dogs).

- Unhealthy Fats: Processed vegetable oils, trans fats (found in fried foods and commercially made goods).

- Sweeteners (Use with Caution): Artificial sweeteners may affect some people with seizures. Consult your doctor before using them.

Chapter 6:

Breakfast Recipes

1. Keto Scrambled Eggs (1 Serving)

Ingredients:

- 2 large eggs

- 1 tablespoon unsalted butter

- Salt and pepper to taste

- Optional additions: Chopped chives, shredded cheese (cheddar, mozzarella)

Preparation:

1. Whisk the eggs in a bowl.

2. Melt the butter in a non-stick pan over medium heat.

3. Pour the egg mixture into the pan and let it cook for a minute, undisturbed.

4. Gently nudge the cooked egg from the edges towards the center of the pan with a spatula, allowing the uncooked egg to flow underneath.

5. Continue cooking, stirring occasionally, until the eggs reach your desired level of doneness (soft scrambled, medium scrambled, or well-done).

6. Season with salt and pepper to taste.

7. Serve immediately with your desired optional additions.

Nutritional Value (estimated):

- Calories: 200

- Fat: 14g

- Protein: 12g

- Net Carbs: 1g

Time: 5 minutes

2. Bacon and Spinach Frittata
(2-3 Servings)

Ingredients:

- 8 large eggs

- 1/4 cup heavy cream

- 1/4 cup shredded cheddar cheese

- 4 slices bacon, cooked and chopped

- 2 cups spinach, roughly chopped

- 1/4 cup chopped onion (optional)

- Salt and pepper to taste

Preparation:

1. Preheat oven to 375°F (190°C).

2. In a bowl, whisk together eggs, heavy cream, and half of the shredded cheese. Season with salt and pepper.

3. In a 10-inch oven-safe skillet, cook the chopped onion (if using) over medium heat until softened.

4. Add the chopped spinach and cook until wilted.

5. Spread the spinach evenly in the skillet.

6. Top with the cooked bacon and pour the egg mixture over the top.

7. Sprinkle the remaining shredded cheese on top.

8. Bake for 20-25 minutes, or until the center is set and a toothpick inserted comes out clean.

9. Let cool slightly before slicing and serving.

Nutritional Value per Serving (estimated):

- Calories: 350

- Fat: 28g

- Protein: 20g

- Net Carbs: 5g

Time: 30 minutes

3. Avocado and Smoked Salmon Plate (1 Serving)

Ingredients:

- 1 ripe avocado, halved, pitted, and sliced

- 3 ounces smoked salmon

- 1 tablespoon lemon juice (optional)

- Pinch of sea salt and freshly ground black pepper

- Optional additions: Chopped chives, a dollop of sour cream

Preparation:

1. Arrange the avocado slices on a plate.

2. Top with smoked salmon.

3. Drizzle with lemon juice (if using) and season with salt and pepper to taste.

4. Garnish with chopped chives and a dollop of sour cream (optional).

Nutritional Value (estimated):

- Calories: 350

- Fat: 28g

- Protein: 20g

- Net Carbs: 5g

Time: 5 minutes

Tips:

- Feel free to adjust the portion sizes based on your individual needs and preferences.

- Use a rubber spatula to prevent sticking when cooking scrambled eggs.

- Experiment with different types of cheese and vegetables in your frittata.

- Leftover frittata can be stored in the refrigerator for up to 3 days and reheated for a quick and easy meal prep option.

- Choose high-quality smoked salmon for the best flavor in the avocado and smoked salmon plate.

Chapter 7:

Lunch Recipes

1. Chicken Caesar Salad (1 Serving)

Classic Caesar Salad Ingredients (to modify):

- Romaine lettuce hearts, chopped

- Grilled chicken breast, sliced

- Caesar salad dressing (**high carb!**)

- Parmesan cheese

- Croutons (**high carb!**)

Keto-Friendly Caesar Salad Ingredients:

- Romaine lettuce hearts, chopped

- Grilled chicken breast, sliced

- Caesar dressing (see recipe below)

- Parmesan cheese

- Sliced cherry tomatoes (optional)

- Chopped avocado (optional)

Keto Caesar Dressing:

- 1/4 cup mayonnaise

- 1/4 cup sour cream

- 1 tablespoon lemon juice

- 1 teaspoon Dijon mustard

- 1 clove garlic, minced

- 1 anchovy fillet (optional, for a stronger umami flavor)

- 1/4 teaspoon Worcestershire sauce

- Salt and pepper to taste

- 1/4 cup grated Parmesan cheese

Preparation:

1. **Dressing:** Combine all dressing ingredients in a blender or food processor until smooth. Season with salt and pepper to taste.

2. **Salad:** In a bowl, toss together romaine lettuce, grilled chicken, parmesan cheese, and any additional toppings you choose.

3. Drizzle with the Caesar dressing and enjoy!

Nutritional Value (estimated):

- Calories: 450

- Fat: 35g

- Protein: 40g

- Net Carbs: 5g (depending on the amount of vegetables added)

Time: 15 minutes (including dressing preparation)

2. Tuna Lettuce Wraps (2 Servings)

Ingredients:

- 2 cans (5 oz each) tuna packed in water, drained

- 1/4 cup mayonnaise

- 1 tablespoon Dijon mustard

- 1 celery stalk, finely chopped

- 1/4 cup red onion, finely chopped

- Salt and pepper to taste

- 4 large romaine lettuce leaves

Preparation:

1. In a bowl, combine tuna, mayonnaise, Dijon mustard, celery, red onion, salt, and pepper.

2. Wash and dry the romaine lettuce leaves.

3. Spoon the tuna mixture onto each lettuce leaf.

4. Wrap the lettuce leaves around the filling and enjoy!

Nutritional Value per Serving (estimated):

- Calories: 300

- Fat: 20g

- Protein: 25g

- Net Carbs: 5g

Time: 10 minutes

3. Egg Salad Stuffed Peppers (2 Servings)

Ingredients:

- 2 large bell peppers, any color

- 4 hard-boiled eggs, chopped

- 1/4 cup mayonnaise

- 1 tablespoon Dijon mustard

- 1 tablespoon chopped celery (optional)

- 1 tablespoon chopped red onion (optional)

- Salt and pepper to taste

- 1/4 cup shredded cheese (optional)

Preparation:

1. Preheat oven to 375°F (190°C).

2. Cut the bell peppers in half, removing the seeds and membranes.

3. In a bowl, combine chopped eggs, mayonnaise, Dijon mustard, celery (if using), red onion (if using), salt, and pepper.

4. Stuff the bell pepper halves with the egg salad mixture.

5. Sprinkle with shredded cheese (if using).

6. Bake for 20-25 minutes, or until the peppers are tender and the cheese is melted (if using).

Nutritional Value per Serving (estimated):

- Calories: 350

- Fat: 25g

- Protein: 20g

- Net Carbs: 8g (depending on the type of pepper used)

Time: 35 minutes

Chapter 8:

Dinner Recipes

1. Grilled Lemon Herb Chicken (2 Servings)

Ingredients:

- 2 boneless, skinless chicken breasts

- 2 tablespoons olive oil

- 1 tablespoon lemon juice

- 1 teaspoon dried oregano

- 1/2 teaspoon dried thyme

- 1/4 teaspoon garlic powder

- Salt and freshly ground black pepper to taste

Preparation:

1. In a bowl, whisk together olive oil, lemon juice, oregano, thyme, garlic powder, salt, and pepper.

2. Place the chicken breasts in a shallow dish and pour the marinade over them. Cover and

refrigerate for at least 30 minutes, or up to 4 hours for deeper flavor.

3. Preheat your grill to medium-high heat.

4. Remove the chicken from the marinade and discard the marinade.

5. Grill the chicken breasts for 5-7 minutes per side, or until cooked through and golden brown.

6. Let the chicken rest for a few minutes before slicing and serving.

Nutritional Value per Serving (estimated):

- Calories: 350

- Fat: 25g

- Protein: 40g

- Net Carbs: 0g

Time: 30 minutes (including marinating time)

2. Beef and Broccoli Stir-Fry (2 Servings)

Ingredients:

- 1 pound ground beef

- 1 tablespoon olive oil

- 1 cup broccoli florets

- 1/2 cup chopped red onion

- 1/4 cup sliced red bell pepper (optional)

- 1/4 cup beef broth

- 1 tablespoon soy sauce (or coconut aminos for a keto-friendly option)

- 1 teaspoon sriracha (optional, for a spicy kick)

- 1/2 teaspoon ground ginger

- Salt and freshly ground black pepper to taste

- Sesame seeds for garnish (optional)

Preparation:

1. Heat olive oil in a large skillet or wok over medium-high heat.

2. Add the ground beef and cook until browned, breaking it up with a spoon as it cooks.

3. Add the broccoli florets, red onion, and bell pepper (if using) to the pan and cook for 3-4 minutes, or until the vegetables are tender-crisp.

4. In a small bowl, whisk together beef broth, soy sauce (or coconut aminos), sriracha (if using), and ginger.

5. Pour the sauce into the pan with the beef and vegetables.

6. Bring to a simmer and cook for 1-2 minutes, or until the sauce thickens slightly.

7. Season with salt and pepper to taste.

8. Serve over cauliflower rice (for a keto-friendly option) or your favorite low-carb noodles.

9. Garnish with sesame seeds (optional).

Nutritional Value per Serving (estimated):

- Calories: 450

- Fat: 30g

- Protein: 35g

- Net Carbs: 5g (depending on the type of noodles used)

Time: 20 minutes

3. Baked Salmon with Asparagus (2 Servings)

Ingredients:

- 2 salmon fillets (6 oz each)

- 1 tablespoon olive oil

- 1 lemon, sliced

- 1 bunch asparagus, trimmed

- Salt and freshly ground black pepper to taste

- Optional additions: Chopped fresh herbs (dill, parsley)

Preparation:

1. Preheat oven to 400°F (200°C).

2. Lightly grease a baking dish.

3. Place the salmon fillets in the prepared baking dish.

4. Drizzle the salmon with olive oil and season with salt and pepper.

5. Top the salmon with lemon slices.

6. Arrange the asparagus spears around the salmon.

7. Bake for 15-20 minutes, or until the salmon is cooked through and flakes easily with a fork.

8. Garnish with chopped fresh herbs (optional) and serve immediately.

Nutritional Value per Serving (estimated):

- Calories: 400

- Fat: 30g

- Protein: 40g

- Net Carbs: 5g

Time: 25 minutes

Chapter 9:

Snack Ideas

1. Cheese and Nut Platter

Ingredients:

- A selection of hard and soft cheeses (cheddar, brie, goat cheese, etc.)

- Sliced almonds, walnuts, pecans, macadamias (or your favorite nut choices)

- Optional additions: Sliced cucumber, cherry tomatoes, olives, sugar-free dark chocolate squares

Preparation:

1. Arrange the cheeses on a platter.

2. Scatter the nuts around the cheeses.

3. Add any of the optional additions you like for a burst of flavor and color.

Tips:

- Choose a variety of cheeses with different textures and flavors to keep things interesting.

- Portion out the nuts beforehand to avoid overindulging.

- Opt for raw, unsalted nuts for the healthiest option.

2. Cucumber Slices with Cream Cheese

This is a simple yet refreshing snack that's perfect for on-the-go.

Ingredients:

- 1 cucumber, sliced into rounds

- 2-3 tablespoons cream cheese, softened

- Optional additions: Chopped fresh herbs (dill, chives), everything bagel seasoning

Preparation:

1. Spread a thin layer of softened cream cheese on each cucumber slice.

2. Sprinkle with your chosen optional additions (if using).

3. Enjoy!

Tips:

- Use a mandoline slicer for perfectly even cucumber slices.

- If the cream cheese is too firm, microwave it for a few seconds to soften it slightly.

- Experiment with different flavors by adding spices or herbs to the cream cheese.

3. Hard-Boiled Eggs

A classic and convenient keto-friendly snack packed with protein and healthy fats.

Ingredients:

- Eggs

Preparation:

1. Place the eggs in a single layer in a saucepan.

2. Cover the eggs with cold water and bring to a boil.

3. Once boiling, remove the pan from the heat and cover it.

4. Let the eggs sit for 10-12 minutes for a medium-cooked yolk. (Adjust time for desired doneness.)

5. Drain the hot water and run cold water over the eggs to stop the cooking process.

6. Peel the eggs and enjoy!

Tips:

- For easier peeling, place the eggs in a bowl of ice water after cooking for a few minutes.

- You can also marinate the hard-boiled eggs in your favorite spices or herbs for added flavor.

- Pre-boil a batch of eggs on Sundays to have a ready-to-go snack throughout the week.

Chapter 10:

Introduction to Balancing Phase

Transitioning from Induction to Ongoing Low-Carb (OLC) in Atkins for Epilepsy:

Reintroducing Carbs Carefully

The initial phase of the Atkins diet for Epilepsy, Induction, is a very low-carb period meant to kickstart ketosis. However, it's not meant to be sustainable long-term. Transitioning to the Ongoing Low-Carb (OLC) phase includes gradually reintroducing certain carbs while maintaining ketosis. Here's a guide to handle this transition safely and effectively:

Signs You're Ready to Move On:

You've achieved and maintained ketosis for at least 2-4 weeks (as proven by blood ketone monitoring or urine test strips under your doctor's guidance).

You've reached your initial weight loss goal (if relevant).

You're having no significant side effects from the Atkins diet.

Important Considerations Before Reintroducing Carbs:

- Do it Gradually: Don't jump back into high-carb foods suddenly. This can disrupt ketosis and possibly trigger seizures. Reintroduce carbs slowly, one food group at a time, in small amounts.

- Work with your Healthcare Professional: They will adjust your carb reintroduction plan based on your individual needs, seizure control, and response to the diet. They can also watch your progress and adjust the plan as needed.

Continue Blood Ketone Monitoring: Monitor your blood ketone levels to ensure you stay in ketosis. Aim for a moderate ketone range as decided by your doctor.

Foods to Gradually Reintroduce:

- Low-Glycemic Fruits: Start with berries like raspberries and strawberries, which are lower in sugar and carbs compared to other fruits.

- Starchy veggies: Reintroduce low-glycemic starchy veggies like sweet potatoes, butternut squash, and turnips in small portions.

- Legumes (Limited): Lentils and chickpeas can be returned in moderation due to their higher fiber content. Consult your doctor for specific suggestions.

- Whole Grains (Limited): Choose whole grains like brown rice or quinoa in small portions, focused on complex carbohydrates.

Foods to Continue Avoiding:

- Sugary Drinks: Soda, juice, sweetened teas, and sports drinks are still off-limits.

- Sugary Fruits: Avoid most fruits except berries in moderation.

- Refined carbs: White bread, pasta, rice, and other refined carbs should still be limited.

- Starchy Vegetables: Potatoes, corn, and peas are still high in carbs and should be avoided or limited.

- Processed Foods: Continue to steer clear of processed snacks, sugary sauces, and unhealthy fats.

Additional Tips:

Focus on Whole, Unprocessed Foods: Prioritize whole, unprocessed foods like veggies, lean protein, and healthy fats.

- Listen to Your Body: Pay attention to how your body responds to reintroduced carbs. If you experience any negative effects like increased seizures, bloating, or fatigue, adjust your carb intake accordingly and contact your doctor.
- Be Patient: Transitioning from Induction to OLC takes time and personalization. Be patient with yourself and focus on making sustainable changes that support your general health and well-being.

Chapter 11:

Breakfast Recipes –

1. Greek Yogurt with Berries and Nuts

Ingredients:

- 1 cup plain Greek yogurt (full-fat)

- 1/4 cup berries (raspberries, strawberries, blueberries)

- 1/4 cup chopped nuts (almonds, walnuts, pecans)

- Optional additions: A drizzle of sugar-free syrup, a sprinkle of cinnamon

Preparation:

1. In a bowl, scoop in your Greek yogurt.

2. Wash and pat dry your berries. Scatter them over the yogurt, creating a beautiful burst of color.

3. Roughly chop your chosen nuts and sprinkle them on top, adding a delightful textural contrast.

4. If desired, drizzle with a sugar-free syrup for a touch of sweetness and finish with a sprinkle of cinnamon for extra warmth.

2. Keto Pancakes with Berries

Ingredients:

- 2 large eggs

- 1/4 cup almond flour

- 1/4 teaspoon baking powder

- 1 tablespoon unsweetened almond milk

- Pinch of salt

- Coconut oil for greasing the pan

- Berries (raspberries, strawberries, blueberries) for serving

Preparation:

1. In a bowl, whisk together eggs, almond flour, baking powder, almond milk, and salt until smooth.

2. Heat a non-stick pan or griddle greased with coconut oil over medium heat.

3. Pour batter into small circles, forming your pancakes.

4. Cook for 2-3 minutes per side, or until golden brown and cooked through.

5. Serve your fluffy keto pancakes with a delightful dollop of whipped cream and a sprinkle of berries.

3. Omelet with Cheese and Vegetables

Ingredients:

- 2 large eggs

- 1 tablespoon milk (whole milk or unsweetened almond milk)

- Pinch of salt and pepper

- 1/4 cup shredded cheese (cheddar, mozzarella, goat cheese)

- 1/2 cup chopped vegetables (spinach, mushrooms, bell peppers, onions)

- Optional additions: Chopped herbs (fresh chives, parsley)

Preparation:

1. In a bowl, whisk together eggs, milk, salt, and pepper.

2. Heat a non-stick pan or skillet greased with butter or cooking spray over medium heat.

3. Pour the egg mixture into the pan and swirl to coat the bottom.

4. As the omelet begins to set, sprinkle your chosen cheese over one half.

5. Add your chopped vegetables to the cheese side.

6. Once cooked through, use a spatula to fold the other half of the omelet over the filling.

7. Garnish with chopped herbs for an extra touch of flavor (optional).

Chapter 12:

Lunch Recipes

1. Cobb Salad with Avocado

Ingredients:

- Romaine lettuce, chopped

- Grilled chicken breast, sliced

- Chopped bacon

- Sliced avocado

- Chopped tomato

- Chopped cucumber

- Crumbled blue cheese (optional)

- Keto-friendly salad dressing (see recipe below)

Keto-Friendly Salad Dressing:

- 1/4 cup olive oil

- 2 tablespoons lemon juice

- 1 tablespoon Dijon mustard

- 1 teaspoon Worcestershire sauce

- Salt and pepper to taste

Preparation:

1. In a bowl, combine chopped romaine lettuce, grilled chicken, bacon, avocado, tomato, and cucumber.

2. Crumble blue cheese over the salad (optional).

3. In a separate bowl, whisk together olive oil, lemon juice, Dijon mustard, Worcestershire sauce, salt, and pepper for your creamy keto-friendly dressing.

4. Toss the salad with the desired amount of dressing and enjoy!

2. Turkey and Cheese Roll-Ups

Ingredients:

- Sliced deli turkey breast

- Cream cheese, softened

- Shredded cheddar cheese

- Chopped spinach or other greens (optional)

- Spices (optional): paprika, garlic powder, onion powder

Preparation:

1. Spread a thin layer of softened cream cheese on each slice of deli turkey.

2. Sprinkle with shredded cheddar cheese and any desired chopped greens (spinach, arugula).

3. Season with paprika, garlic powder, and onion powder for an extra flavor boost (optional).

4. Roll up the turkey slices tightly and secure them with toothpicks (optional).

5. Slice the roll-ups into bite-sized pieces for easy eating.

3. Spinach and Bacon Quiche

Ingredients:

- 1 cup almond flour

- 1/4 cup melted butter

- 1/4 teaspoon salt

- 4 eggs

- 1 cup chopped spinach

- 1/2 cup chopped cooked bacon

- 1/2 cup shredded cheese (cheddar, mozzarella)

- 1/4 cup heavy cream (optional)

- Pinch of nutmeg (optional)

Preparation:

1. Preheat oven to 375°F (190°C).

2. In a bowl, combine almond flour, melted butter, and salt. Press the mixture into the bottom of a pie dish, forming a crust.

3. In a separate bowl, whisk together eggs, spinach, bacon, shredded cheese, heavy cream (if using), and nutmeg (if using).

4. Pour the egg mixture into the prepared almond flour crust.

5. Bake for 30-35 minutes, or until the center is set and a toothpick inserted comes out clean.

6. Let cool slightly before slicing and serving.

Chapter 13:

Dinner Recipes

1. Garlic Butter Shrimp

Ingredients:

- 1 pound raw shrimp, peeled and deveined

- 2 tablespoons butter

- 2 cloves garlic, minced

- Salt and pepper to taste

- Optional additions: Chopped fresh parsley, a squeeze of lemon juice

Preparation:

1. Heat butter in a large skillet over medium heat.

2. Add minced garlic and cook for 30 seconds, until fragrant.

3. Add shrimp and cook for 2-3 minutes per side, or until pink and opaque.

4. Season with salt and pepper to taste.

5. Garnish with chopped fresh parsley and a squeeze of lemon juice (optional).

2. Pork Chops with Green Beans

Ingredients:

- 2 bone-in pork chops

- 1 tablespoon olive oil

- Salt and pepper to taste

- 1 pound fresh green beans, trimmed

- 2 tablespoons butter

Preparation:

1. Preheat oven to 400°F (200°C).

2. Pat the pork chops dry with paper towels. Season generously with salt and pepper.

3. Heat olive oil in a large skillet over medium-high heat. Sear the pork chops for 2-3 minutes per side, for a nice golden brown sear.

4. Transfer the seared pork chops to a baking dish.

5. Toss the green beans with olive oil, salt, and pepper.

6. Arrange the green beans around the pork chops in the baking dish.

7. Dot the top of the pork chops with butter.

8. Bake for 15-20 minutes, or until the pork chops are cooked through and the green beans are tender-crisp.

3. Stuffed Bell Peppers

Ingredients:

- 2 large bell peppers, any color

- 1 pound ground beef

- 1/2 cup chopped onion

- 1/2 cup chopped mushrooms

- 1/4 cup chopped celery (optional)

- 1 clove garlic, minced

- 1/2 cup shredded cheese (cheddar, mozzarella)

- 1/4 cup chopped fresh parsley

- 1/4 cup tomato sauce (optional)

- Salt and pepper to taste

Preparation:

1. Preheat oven to 375°F (190°C).

2. Cut the tops off the bell peppers and remove the seeds and membranes.

3. In a large skillet over medium heat, brown the ground beef. Drain off any excess grease.

4. Add chopped onion, mushrooms, celery (if using), and garlic to the pan. Cook until softened.

5. Stir in the shredded cheese, chopped parsley, and tomato sauce (if using). Season with salt and pepper to taste.

6. Spoon the filling into the prepared bell peppers.

7. Bake for 20-25 minutes, or until the bell peppers are tender and the filling is cooked through.

Chapter 14:

Snack Ideas

1. Almond Flour Crackers.

Ingredients:

- 1 cup almond flour

- 1/4 teaspoon baking powder

- 1/4 teaspoon salt

- 3 tablespoons melted butter or coconut oil

- 1-2 tablespoons water (gradually add)

- Optional additions: Spices (garlic powder, onion powder, Italian seasoning), sesame seeds

Preparation:

1. Preheat oven to 350°F (175°C).

2. In a bowl, whisk together almond flour, baking powder, and salt.

3. Add melted butter or coconut oil and mix until crumbly.

4. Gradually add water, 1 tablespoon at a time, until a dough forms that is slightly sticky but can be handled.

5. Roll out the dough on a parchment-lined baking sheet to a thin layer (about 1/4 inch thickness).

6. Use a pizza cutter or knife to score the dough into desired cracker shapes. Sprinkle with any chosen optional additions.

7. Bake for 10-12 minutes, or until golden brown and crisp around the edges.

8. Let cool completely before storing in an airtight container.

Nutritional Value (per serving, about 4 crackers):

- Calories: 120

- Fat: 9g

- Protein: 4g

- Net Carbs: 2g

Time: 30 minutes (including baking time)

2. Celery Sticks with Almond Butter

Ingredients:

- Celery sticks

- Almond butter (unsweetened)

Preparation:

1. Wash and cut celery stalks into bite-sized pieces.

2. Spread a generous dollop of almond butter on each celery stick.

Nutritional Value (per serving, 2 celery sticks with 2 tablespoons almond butter):

- Calories: 220

- Fat: 16g

- Protein: 6g

- Net Carbs: 5g (depending on the almond butter brand)

Time: 2 minutes

3. Keto Fat Bombs

Ingredients:

- 1/2 cup unsweetened almond butter

- 1/4 cup melted coconut oil

- 2 tablespoons unsweetened cocoa powder

- 2 tablespoons powdered sweetener (suitable for baking)

- Pinch of salt

- Optional additions: Vanilla extract, chopped nuts, shredded coconut

Preparation:

1. In a bowl, combine almond butter, melted coconut oil, cocoa powder, powdered sweetener, and salt. Mix until well combined.

2. Fold in any chosen optional additions (vanilla extract, chopped nuts, shredded coconut).

3. Line a mini muffin tin with silicone liners or parchment paper.

4. Spoon the mixture into the prepared muffin tin, filling each mold about ¾ full.

5. Place the tin in the freezer for at least 2 hours, or until firm.

Nutritional Value (per serving, 1 fat bomb):

- Calories: 200

- Fat: 18g

- Protein: 2g

- Net Carbs: 2g (depending on the powdered sweetener used)

Time: 2 hours (mostly freezing time) + 5 minutes preparation

Chapter 15:

Introduction to Fine-Tuning Phase

Identifying Your Personal Carbohydrate Tolerance:

A Guide for Continued Weight Loss and Health Benefits

While there isn't a one-size-fits-all method, identifying your personal carbohydrate tolerance can be a powerful tool for maintaining weight loss and maximizing health benefits on a low-carb diet. Here's a breakdown to help you handle this process:

Why Identify Your Tolerance?

Sustainable Weight Loss: Finding your sweet spot for carbs allows you to gradually reintroduce some carbs while still keeping a calorie deficit, promoting long-term weight management.

- Improved Energy Levels: Some people suffer low energy on very low-carb diets. Identifying your tolerance can help you find the balance between ketosis and proper energy levels.

- Reduced Cravings: Extreme carb reduction can lead to cravings. Knowing your tolerance allows for occasional higher-carb choices, reducing cravings and making your diet more sustainable.

- Personalized Approach: Everyone's body reacts differently to carbs. Finding your tolerance helps tailor the diet to your unique needs and improve health benefits.

Methods for Identifying Your Tolerance:

Track Your Carbs and Weight: Start by keeping a thorough food diary, logging your carb intake and weight fluctuations. Gradually increase carb intake in small increments (10-20 grams per day) while watching your weight. When you see a consistent weight increase or a decrease in energy levels, that might suggest reaching your tolerance limit.

Biofeedback Tools: Ketone testing strips or blood ketone meters can be used to measure your ketone levels. Remember, ketosis isn't the only sign of success. Focus on finding a balance between healthy ketone levels and general well-being.

Consult a Healthcare Professional: A doctor, registered dietitian, or other qualified healthcare worker can help you personalize your approach, taking into account your individual health goals and medical history.

Maintaining Weight Loss and Health Benefits:

- Focus on Whole Foods: Prioritize nutrient-dense, whole foods like veggies, lean protein, and healthy fats.

- Mindful Eating: Practice mindful eating methods, paying attention to hunger and satiety cues to avoid overeating.

- Physical Activity: Regular exercise is important for weight management and overall health. Aim for at least 150 minutes of moderate-intensity exercise per week.

- Listen to Your Body: Pay attention to how you feel after resuming certain carbs. If you experience negative effects like bloating or fatigue, change your intake accordingly.

Important Considerations:

- Don't Rush: Identifying your tolerance takes time and practice. Be patient and change your carb intake gradually.

- Individuality: What works for one person might not work for another. Don't compare your tolerance to others on the same diet.

- Freedom: Allow for some freedom in your carb intake. Occasional higher-carb meals can be part of a healthy diet.

Additional Tips:

- Focus on Quality Over Quantity: Opt for low-glycemic carbs that have a minimal effect on blood sugar levels, such as non-starchy vegetables and berries.

- Fiber is Your Friend: Fiber helps control digestion and keeps you feeling fuller for longer. Prioritize high-fiber carbs like whole grains and beans (in moderation).

Chapter 16:

Breakfast Recipes

1. Chia Seed Pudding

Ingredients (Basic Recipe):

- 1/4 cup chia seeds

- 1 cup unsweetened nut milk (almond milk, coconut milk)

- 1-2 tablespoons sweetener (suitable for baking, like erythritol or stevia)

- Optional additions: Vanilla extract, cinnamon, cocoa powder, chopped nuts, berries

Preparation:

1. In a bowl or jar, combine chia seeds, nut milk, and sweetener.

2. Stir in any chosen optional additions (vanilla extract, cinnamon, cocoa powder, chopped nuts).

3. Cover the container and refrigerate overnight, or for at least 4 hours, allowing the chia seeds to absorb the liquid and thicken.

4. In the morning, give it a stir and enjoy!

Nutritional Value (per serving, basic recipe):

- Calories: 250

- Fat: 14g

- Protein: 4g

- Net Carbs: 5g (depending on the sweetener used)

Time: 5 minutes prep + overnight refrigeration

2. Low-Carb Smoothies

Ingredients (Sample Recipe):

- 1 cup unsweetened almond milk

- 1 scoop protein powder (unflavored or keto-friendly flavor)

- 1/2 cup frozen spinach

- 1/4 cup berries (raspberries, blueberries, strawberries)

- 1 tablespoon almond butter

- Handful of ice cubes (optional)

Preparation:

1. Blend all ingredients together in a high-powered blender until smooth and creamy.

2. Add ice cubes for a thicker consistency (optional).

Nutritional Value (per serving, sample recipe):

- Calories: 300

- Fat: 18g

- Protein: 20g

- Net Carbs: 5g (depending on the protein powder used)

Time: 5 minutes

3. Keto Muffins

Ingredients (Basic Recipe):

- 1 cup almond flour

- 1/4 cup melted coconut oil

- 3 large eggs

- 1/4 cup unsweetened almond milk

- 2 tablespoons sweetener (suitable for baking)

- 1 teaspoon baking powder

- 1/2 teaspoon salt

- Optional additions: Vanilla extract, cinnamon, chopped nuts, berries

Preparation:

1. Preheat oven to 350°F (175°C).

2. In a bowl, whisk together almond flour, baking powder, and salt.

3. In a separate bowl, whisk together melted coconut oil, eggs, almond milk, and sweetener.

4. Combine the wet and dry ingredients, mixing until just combined.

5. Fold in any chosen optional additions (vanilla extract, cinnamon, chopped nuts, berries).

6. Spoon the batter into greased muffin tins.

7. Bake for 15-20 minutes, or until a toothpick inserted into the center comes out clean.

Nutritional Value (per serving, 1 muffin):

- Calories: 280

- Fat: 20g

- Protein: 6g

- Net Carbs: 3g (depending on the sweetener used)

Time: 1 hour (including baking time) + 10 minutes prep

Chapter 17:

Lunch Recipes

1. Grilled Chicken and Avocado Salad

Ingredients:

- Grilled chicken breast (grilled beforehand, about 1 breast per serving)

- 1 large avocado, sliced

- 2 cups mixed greens (arugula, spinach, romaine)

- 1/2 cup cherry tomatoes, halved

- 1/4 cup crumbled feta cheese (optional)

- Keto-friendly salad dressing (see recipe below)

Keto-Friendly Salad Dressing:

- 1/4 cup olive oil

- 2 tablespoons lemon juice

- 1 tablespoon Dijon mustard

- 1 teaspoon Worcestershire sauce

- Salt and pepper to taste

Preparation:

1. Assemble the salad by placing mixed greens on a plate.

2. Top with sliced grilled chicken breast, avocado, cherry tomatoes, and crumbled feta cheese (if using).

3. Drizzle with your desired amount of keto-friendly salad dressing.

Nutritional Value (per serving, without feta cheese):

- Calories: 450

- Fat: 30g

- Protein: 40g

- Net Carbs: 5g

Time: 10 minutes (assuming chicken is already grilled)

2. Cauliflower Rice Sushi

Ingredients:

- 1 cup riced cauliflower (can be purchased pre-riced or riced at home)

- 1 tablespoon rice vinegar

- 1 tablespoon sesame oil

- 1 sheet nori seaweed

- Keto-friendly sushi fillings (sliced avocado, cucumber, cooked salmon, cream cheese)

- Optional additions: Wasabi paste, pickled ginger

Preparation:

1. In a bowl, combine riced cauliflower, rice vinegar, and sesame oil. Mix well and set aside for 5 minutes.

2. Place a sheet of nori seaweed on a bamboo mat (if using). Spread a thin layer of cauliflower rice over half of the nori, leaving a border at the top.

3. Add your chosen keto-friendly fillings along the center of the rice.

4. With the help of the bamboo mat, tightly roll up the nori, starting from the filled side and using the border to seal the roll.

5. Slice the roll into bite-sized pieces and serve with optional wasabi paste and pickled ginger.

Nutritional Value (per serving, 1 roll with salmon and avocado):

- Calories: 250

- Fat: 15g

- Protein: 20g

- Net Carbs: 5g

Time: 20 minutes

3. Zucchini Noodles with Pesto

Ingredients:

- 2 zucchinis, spiralized into noodles

- 1/2 cup pesto (homemade or store-bought keto-friendly pesto)

- Cherry tomatoes, halved (optional)

- Chopped fresh basil (optional)

Preparation:

1. Using a spiralizer, spiralize the zucchinis into noodles.

2. Heat a large skillet over medium heat. Add the zucchini noodles and cook for 2-3 minutes, or until slightly softened.

3. Stir in the pesto and cook for another minute, until heated through.

4. Divide the zucchini noodles with pesto between plates.

5. Top with cherry tomatoes and chopped fresh basil (optional).

Nutritional Value (per serving, with homemade pesto):

- Calories: 300

- Fat: 20g

- Protein: 8g

- Net Carbs: 7g (depending on the pesto recipe)

Time: 15 minutes

Chapter 18:

Dinner Recipes

1. Herb-Crusted Lamb Chops

Ingredients:

- 4 bone-in lamb chops

- 2 tablespoons olive oil

- 1 tablespoon Dijon mustard

- 1 tablespoon chopped fresh rosemary

- 1 tablespoon chopped fresh thyme

- 1/2 teaspoon garlic powder

- 1/4 teaspoon salt

- 1/4 teaspoon black pepper

Preparation:

1. Preheat oven to 400°F (200°C).

2. In a bowl, whisk together olive oil, Dijon mustard, rosemary, thyme, garlic powder, salt, and pepper.

3. Pat the lamb chops dry with paper towels. Brush both sides generously with the herb mixture.

4. Heat a large oven-safe skillet over medium-high heat. Sear the lamb chops for 2-3 minutes per side, for a nice golden brown sear.

5. Transfer the skillet with the seared lamb chops to the preheated oven and bake for 10-12 minutes for medium-rare, or until desired doneness.

6. Let the lamb chops rest for a few minutes before serving.

Nutritional Value (per serving, 1 lamb chop):

- Calories: 400

- Fat: 30g

- Protein: 35g

- Net Carbs: 0g

Time: 30 minutes (including baking time)

2. Beef and Cauliflower Shepherd's Pie

Ingredients:

- 1 pound ground beef

- 1 onion, chopped

- 2 cloves garlic, minced

- 1 cup chopped mushrooms

- 1 cup chopped celery

- 1/2 cup beef broth

- 1 (14.5 oz) can diced tomatoes, undrained

- 1 tablespoon tomato paste

- 1 teaspoon dried thyme

- 1/2 teaspoon dried rosemary

- Salt and pepper to taste

- 1 head of cauliflower, riced (can be purchased pre-riced or riced at home)

- 1/2 cup shredded cheddar cheese (optional)

Preparation:

1. Preheat oven to 375°F (190°C).

2. In a large skillet over medium heat, brown the ground beef. Drain off any excess grease.

3. Add onion, garlic, mushrooms, and celery to the pan. Cook for 5 minutes, or until softened.

4. Stir in beef broth, diced tomatoes, tomato paste, thyme, rosemary, salt, and pepper. Bring to a simmer and cook for 10 minutes.

5. Transfer the meat mixture to a baking dish.

6. In a separate pot, steam the riced cauliflower for 5-7 minutes, or until tender-crisp. Drain any excess moisture.

7. Season the cauliflower rice with salt and pepper (optional).

8. Spread the cauliflower rice over the meat mixture in the baking dish.

9. Top with shredded cheddar cheese (optional).

10. Bake for 15-20 minutes, or until the cheese is melted and bubbly (if using).

Nutritional Value (per serving):

- Calories: 450

- Fat: 35g

- Protein: 30g

- Net Carbs: 8g (depending on the amount of cauliflower used)

Time: 1 hour

3. Lemon Garlic Butter Scallops

Ingredients:

- 1 pound sea scallops

- 2 tablespoons butter

- 2 tablespoons olive oil

- 2 cloves garlic, minced

- 1 tablespoon lemon juice

- 1/4 cup chopped fresh parsley

- Salt and pepper to taste

Preparation:

1. Pat the scallops dry with paper towels. Season generously with salt and pepper.

2. Heat a large skillet over medium-high heat. Add olive oil and butter.

3. Once the butter is melted and foaming, carefully add the scallops. Sear for 2-3 minutes per side, or until golden brown and cooked through.

4. Add garlic and lemon juice to the pan and cook

Chapter 19:

Snack Ideas

1. Veggie Chips

Ingredients:

- 2 cups thinly sliced vegetables (zucchini, eggplant, kale, bell peppers)

- 1 tablespoon olive oil

- 1/2 teaspoon dried oregano

- 1/2 teaspoon garlic powder

- 1/4 teaspoon paprika

- Salt and pepper to taste

Preparation:

1. Preheat oven to 200°F (93°C).

2. In a bowl, toss the sliced vegetables with olive oil, oregano, garlic powder, paprika, salt, and pepper.

3. Arrange the vegetables in a single layer on a baking sheet lined with parchment paper.

4. Bake for 45-60 minutes, or until the vegetables are crispy and dry, flipping them halfway through baking.

5. Let the chips cool completely before storing in an airtight container.

Nutritional Value (per serving, about 1 cup chips):

- Calories: 70

- Fat: 5g

- Protein: 2g

- Net Carbs: 5g (depending on the vegetables used)

Time: 1-1.5 hours (including baking time)

2. Spiced Nuts

Ingredients:

- 1 cup raw nuts (almonds, pecans, walnuts, macadamia nuts)

- 1 tablespoon melted coconut oil

- 1/2 teaspoon ground cinnamon

- 1/4 teaspoon chili powder (optional)

- 1/4 teaspoon smoked paprika (optional)

- Salt to taste

Preparation:

1. Preheat oven to 300°F (149°C).

2. In a bowl, toss the nuts with melted coconut oil, cinnamon, chili powder (if using), smoked paprika (if using), and salt.

3. Spread the nuts on a baking sheet lined with parchment paper.

4. Bake for 10-12 minutes, stirring occasionally, or until fragrant and golden brown.

5. Let the nuts cool completely before storing in an airtight container.

Nutritional Value (per serving, 1/4 cup nuts):

- Calories: 180

- Fat: 15g

- Protein: 6g

- Net Carbs: 2g (depending on the nut variety)

Time: 30 minutes (including baking time)

3. Chocolate Avocado Mousse

Ingredients:

- 2 ripe avocados, pitted and peeled

- 1/4 cup unsweetened cocoa powder

- 1/4 cup powdered sweetener (suitable for baking, like erythritol or stevia)

- 1/4 cup unsweetened almond milk

- 1 teaspoon vanilla extract

- Pinch of salt

Preparation:

1. In a blender or food processor, combine avocados, cocoa powder, powdered sweetener, almond milk, vanilla extract, and salt.

2. Blend until smooth and creamy, scraping down the sides as needed.

3. Divide the mousse between serving bowls and enjoy immediately, or chill for a thicker consistency.

Nutritional Value (per serving):

- Calories: 300

- Fat: 25g

- Protein: 4g

- Net Carbs: 5g (depending on the powdered sweetener used)

Time: 10 minutes

Chapter 20:

Introduction to Maintenance Phase

Benefits of Flexible Carb Intake:

- Improved Sustainability: A more relaxed attitude to carbs can make the diet feel less restrictive and easier to stick with in the long run.

- Enhanced Social Life: Occasional higher-carb meals allow you to enjoy social events and dining experiences without feeling overly restricted.

- Nutrient Diversity: Strategic inclusion of some carb-rich fruits and vegetables adds important vitamins, minerals, and fiber to your diet.

- Improved Metabolic Health: Carefully planned higher-carb days can help keep metabolic flexibility, which may be beneficial for overall health.

Tips for Flexible Carb Intake on Keto

- **Identify Your Tolerance:** Start by tracking your carb intake and weight fluctuations to understand how your body responds to different carb levels.

- **Plan "Carb-Up" Days (Strategically):** Consider incorporating carefully timed higher-carb days, like before or after intense workouts, to replenish glycogen stores and support performance.

- **Focus on Whole Foods:** Prioritize low-glycemic carbs like non-starchy vegetables and berries over processed carbs when adding them.

- **Mindful Eating:** Practice mindful eating during all meals, focusing on hunger and fullness cues to avoid overeating, even on higher-carb days.

- **Listen to Your Body:** Pay attention to how you feel after resuming certain carbs. Adjust your method based on your individual experience (e.g., bloating, fatigue).

- **Seek Guidance:** Consider consulting a registered dietitian or healthcare professional to develop a personalized flexible keto approach that fits with your goals and health needs.

❀Here's an example of an open approach:

❀ Weekdays: Maintain a stricter keto diet with moderate carb intake (20-50g per day).

❀ Weekends: Allow for one or two higher-carb meals (around 75-100g per day) but favor whole food sources like fruits, starchy vegetables, or whole grains.

Chapter 21:

Breakfast Recipes

1. Mixed Berry Smoothie Bowl

Ingredients:

- 1 cup frozen mixed berries (blueberries, raspberries, strawberries)

- 1/2 cup unsweetened almond milk

- 1/4 cup plain Greek yogurt (optional, for added protein)

- 1 tablespoon chia seeds

- Toppings (granola, chopped nuts, sliced banana)

Preparation:

1. Blend the frozen berries, almond milk, and Greek yogurt (if using) until smooth and creamy.

2. Pour the smoothie mixture into a bowl.

3. Top with your favorite toppings like granola, chopped nuts, or sliced banana.

Nutritional Value (per serving, without toppings):

- Calories: 200

- Fat: 5g

- Protein: 8g (with Greek yogurt)

- Net Carbs: 15g (depending on the berry blend)

Time: 5 minutes

2. Keto Granola

Ingredients:

- 1 cup chopped nuts (almonds, pecans, walnuts)

- 1/2 cup unsweetened shredded coconut

- 1/4 cup sunflower seeds

- 2 tablespoons melted butter or coconut oil

- 1/4 cup granulated sugar substitute (suitable for baking)

- 1 teaspoon ground cinnamon

- Pinch of salt

Preparation:

1. Preheat oven to 300°F (149°C).

2. In a bowl, combine nuts, coconut, and sunflower seeds.

3. In a separate bowl, whisk together melted butter or coconut oil, sugar substitute, cinnamon, and salt.

4. Pour the wet ingredients over the dry ingredients and mix well.

5. Spread the mixture on a baking sheet lined with parchment paper.

6. Bake for 15-20 minutes, or until golden brown, stirring occasionally.

7. Let the granola cool completely before storing in an airtight container.

Nutritional Value (per serving, 1/4 cup):

- Calories: 250

- Fat: 18g

- Protein: 4g

- Net Carbs: 5g (depending on the sugar substitute used)

Time: 30 minutes (including baking time)

3. Eggs Benedict with Hollandaise Sauce

Ingredients:

- 2 English muffins (or low-carb alternative)

- 4 slices Canadian bacon

- 4 eggs

- Hollandaise sauce (recipe below)

Hollandaise Sauce Ingredients:

- 3 egg yolks

- 1 tablespoon lemon juice

- 1/4 cup melted butter

- Pinch of salt

- Pinch of cayenne pepper (optional)

Preparation:

1. Poach the eggs: Bring a pot of water to a simmer. Crack each egg into a separate small bowl or ramekin. Once the water simmers, gently swirl the water to create a vortex. Carefully slide each egg into the center of the vortex and cook for 3-4 minutes, or until desired doneness.

2. Toast the English muffins (or prepare your low-carb alternative).

3. While the eggs are poaching, prepare the hollandaise sauce. (see instructions below)

4. Assemble the Eggs Benedict: Place a toasted English muffin half on a plate. Top with Canadian bacon, a poached egg, and hollandaise sauce.

Hollandaise Sauce Instructions:

1. In a blender or food processor, combine egg yolks, lemon juice, salt, and cayenne pepper (if using). Blend for 30 seconds, until frothy and light yellow.

2. With the blender running on low speed, slowly drizzle in the melted butter until the sauce is thick and creamy.

Nutritional Value (per serving, with English muffins):

- Calories: 700 (depending on the hollandaise sauce)

- Fat: 50g

- Protein: 25g

- Net Carbs: 40g

Chapter 22:

Lunch Recipes

1. Quinoa and Avocado Salad

Ingredients:

- 1 cup cooked quinoa

- 1 ripe avocado, diced

- 1/2 cup cherry tomatoes, halved

- 1/4 cup crumbled feta cheese (optional)

- 1/4 cup chopped red onion

- 1 tablespoon chopped fresh cilantro

- Lime juice (to taste)

- Olive oil (to taste)

- Salt and pepper to taste

Preparation:

1. In a bowl, combine cooked quinoa, diced avocado, cherry tomatoes, feta cheese (if using), red onion, and chopped cilantro.

2. Drizzle with lime juice and olive oil to taste.

3. Season with salt and pepper to taste.

Nutritional Value (per serving, without feta cheese):

- Calories: 350

- Fat: 15g

- Protein: 8g

- Net Carbs: 30g (depending on the quinoa variety)

Time: 15 minutes (assuming quinoa is already cooked)

2. Chicken and Zoodle Soup

Ingredients:

- 4 cups chicken broth

- 2 boneless, skinless chicken breasts, cooked and shredded

- 2 zucchini, spiralized into noodles (zoodles)

- 1 onion, chopped

- 2 cloves garlic, minced

- 1 teaspoon dried oregano

- 1/2 teaspoon dried thyme

- Salt and pepper to taste

- Chopped fresh parsley (optional, for garnish)

Preparation:

1. In a large pot, heat the chicken broth over medium heat.

2. Add the chopped onion and garlic, and cook until softened, about 5 minutes.

3. Stir in the shredded chicken, oregano, thyme, salt, and pepper.

4. Bring the soup to a simmer.

5. Add the spiralized zucchini noodles and cook for 2-3 minutes, or until tender-crisp.

6. Taste and adjust seasonings as needed.

7. Serve hot, garnished with chopped fresh parsley (optional).

Nutritional Value (per serving):

- Calories: 300

- Fat: 10g

- Protein: 30g

- Net Carbs: 5g (depending on the amount of zucchini used)

Time: 30 minutes

3. Eggplant Lasagna

Ingredients:

- 1 large eggplant, sliced into thin rounds

- 1 pound ground beef

- 1 onion, chopped

- 2 cloves garlic, minced

- 1 (14.5 oz) can diced tomatoes, undrained

- 1 tablespoon tomato paste

- 1 teaspoon dried oregano

- 1/2 teaspoon dried basil

- 1 cup shredded mozzarella cheese

- 1/4 cup grated Parmesan cheese

- Salt and pepper to taste

Preparation:

1. Preheat oven to 375°F (190°C).

2. In a large skillet over medium heat, brown the ground beef. Drain off any excess grease.

3. Add the chopped onion and garlic to the pan, and cook until softened.

4. Stir in the diced tomatoes, tomato paste, oregano, and basil. Bring to a simmer and cook for 10 minutes.

5. Season with salt and pepper to taste.

6. In a shallow baking dish, layer the sliced eggplant (arrange slightly overlapping) followed by the meat sauce, and then sprinkle with mozzarella cheese.

7. Repeat the layering process, ending with a top layer of eggplant and mozzarella cheese.

8. Sprinkle the top with Parmesan cheese.

9. Bake for 30-35 minutes, or until the eggplant is tender and the cheese is melted and bubbly.

Nutritional Value (per serving):

- Calories: 450

- Fat: 30g

- Protein: 35g

- Net Carbs: 8g

Chapter 23:

Dinner Recipes

1. Baked Cod with Lemon and Herbs

Ingredients:

- 2 cod fillets

- 2 tablespoons olive oil

- 1 tablespoon lemon juice

- 1 teaspoon chopped fresh rosemary

- 1/2 teaspoon dried thyme

- Salt and pepper to taste

Preparation:

1. Preheat oven to 400°F (200°C).

2. In a shallow baking dish, toss cod fillets with olive oil, lemon juice, rosemary, thyme, salt, and pepper.

3. Bake for 10-12 minutes, or until the cod flakes easily with a fork.

Nutritional Value (per serving):

*   Calories: 350

*   Fat: 25g

*   Protein: 40g

*   Net Carbs: 0g

Time: 15 minutes (including baking time)

2. Beef Stroganoff with Cauliflower Mash

Ingredients:

*   **For the Beef Stroganoff:**

    o   1 pound beef sirloin, cut into thin strips

    o   1 tablespoon olive oil

    o   1 onion, chopped

    o   2 cloves garlic, minced

    o   1 cup sliced mushrooms

- o 1 (10.5 oz) can condensed cream of mushroom soup (unsweetened keto-friendly version)

- o 1/2 cup beef broth

- o 1/4 cup dry sherry (optional)

- o 1 tablespoon Dijon mustard

- o Salt and pepper to taste

- **For the Cauliflower Mash:**

  - o 1 head of cauliflower, riced (can be purchased pre-riced or riced at home)

  - o 1/4 cup heavy cream

  - o 2 tablespoons butter

  - o Salt and pepper to taste

Preparation:

1. **Make the Cauliflower Mash:** In a pot, steam the riced cauliflower for 5-7 minutes, or until tender-crisp. Drain any excess moisture.

2. In a separate pan, melt butter over medium heat. Add the mashed cauliflower and heavy cream.

Season with salt and pepper to taste. Mash with a potato masher or blend until smooth (optional). Set aside.

3. **Prepare the Beef Stroganoff:** Heat olive oil in a large skillet over medium-high heat. Sear the beef strips for 2-3 minutes, or until browned.

4. Add the chopped onion and garlic to the pan, and cook until softened.

5. Stir in the sliced mushrooms and cook for an additional minute.

6. Pour in the cream of mushroom soup, beef broth, sherry (if using), and Dijon mustard.

7. Bring the sauce to a simmer and cook for 5-7 minutes, or until slightly thickened. Season with salt and pepper to taste.

8. Serve the beef stroganoff over a bed of cauliflower mash.

Nutritional Value (per serving):

- Calories: 500

- Fat: 35g

- Protein: 40g

- Net Carbs: 5g (depending on the cauliflower mash)

Time: 45 minutes

3. Chicken Alfredo with Spaghetti Squash

This dish offers a delicious low-carb alternative to traditional pasta Alfredo.

Ingredients:

- 1 spaghetti squash, halved and seeds removed

- 1 tablespoon olive oil

- 1 pound boneless, skinless chicken breasts, cooked and shredded

- 1 onion, chopped

- 2 cloves garlic, minced

- 1 cup heavy cream

- 1/2 cup grated Parmesan cheese

- 1/4 cup shredded mozzarella cheese

- 1/4 cup chopped fresh parsley

- Salt and pepper to taste

Preparation:

1. Preheat oven to 400°F (200°C).

2. Brush the cut sides of the spaghetti squash halves with olive oil. Season with salt and pepper.

3. Place the squash halves face down on a baking sheet. Roast for 30-40 minutes, or until tender-crisp and easily shreddable with a fork.

4. While the squash roasts, cook the shredded chicken (if not already cooked).

5. In a large skillet over medium heat, heat olive oil. Add the chopped onion and garlic, and cook until softened.

6. Stir in the shredded chicken and cook for an additional minute or two.

7. Pour in the heavy cream and bring to a simmer. Reduce heat to low and simmer for 5 minutes.

8. Remove the pan from heat and stir in the grated Parmesan cheese and shredded mozzarella cheese until melted and sauce is creamy. Season with salt and pepper to taste.

9. Once the spaghetti squash is cooked, remove it from the oven and use a fork to scrape out the flesh, creating spaghetti-like strands.

6. 10. Divide the spaghetti squash strands between plates and top with the creamy chicken Alfredo sauce.
7. 11. Garnish with chopped fresh parsley (optional).

Nutritional Value (per serving):

- Calories: 550

- Fat: 40g

- Protein: 45g

- Net Carbs: 10g (depending on the spaghetti squash)

Time: 1 hour

Chapter 24:

Snack Ideas

1. Trail Mix with Dark Chocolate

Ingredients:

- 1 cup raw nuts (almonds, cashews, walnuts, pecans)

- 1/2 cup dried fruit (raisins, cranberries, cherries)

- 1/4 cup dark chocolate chips (at least 70% cacao)

- 1/4 cup roasted seeds (pumpkin seeds, sunflower seeds)

- Optional additions: shredded coconut, whole-grain cereal squares

Preparation:

1. In a bowl, combine all the ingredients.

2. Store in an airtight container for easy on-the-go snacking.

Tips:

- Adjust the nut, dried fruit, and chocolate chip ratios to your preference.

- Consider toasting the nuts for added flavor.

- Pre-portion the trail mix into individual bags for convenient snacking.

Nutritional Value (per 1/4 cup serving):

- Calories: 200

- Fat: 12g

- Protein: 5g

- Net Carbs: 15g (depending on the dried fruit used)

2. Coconut Yogurt with Berries

Ingredients:

- 1 cup unsweetened coconut yogurt

- 1/2 cup fresh berries (blueberries, raspberries, strawberries)

- Optional additions: granola, chopped nuts, chia seeds, drizzle of honey

Preparation:

1. In a bowl, combine coconut yogurt and fresh berries.

2. Top with your favorite optional ingredients for added texture and flavor.

Tips:

- Choose unsweetened coconut yogurt and add your own natural sweetener like honey or maple syrup for portion-controlled sweetness.

- Frozen berries can be used instead of fresh, but thaw them slightly before adding them to the yogurt.

Nutritional Value (per serving, with no added ingredients):

- Calories: 150

- Fat: 7g

- Protein: 5g

- Net Carbs: 10g (depending on the berries used)

3. Almond Butter Protein Balls

Ingredients:

- 1 cup rolled oats

- 1/2 cup unsweetened almond butter

- 1/4 cup honey or maple syrup

- 1/4 cup chia seeds

- 1/4 cup chopped nuts (optional)

- Pinch of salt

Preparation:

1. In a large bowl, combine rolled oats, almond butter, honey or maple syrup, chia seeds, chopped nuts (if using), and salt.

2. Mix well until everything is well incorporated and the mixture holds its shape when pressed together.

3. Roll the mixture into bite-sized balls using your hands.

4. Store the protein balls in an airtight container in the refrigerator for up to a week.

Tips:

- Substitute almond butter with other nut butters like peanut butter or cashew butter.

- You can add shredded coconut, dried fruit, or dark chocolate chips for additional flavor variations.

Nutritional Value (per 1 ball):

- Calories: 200

- Fat: 10g

- Protein: 5g

- Net Carbs: 20g (depending on the type of sweetener used)

Chapter 25:

Desserts and Treats

1. Keto Cheesecake

Ingredients:

- **For the Crust:**

    o   1 cup almond flour

    o   1/4 cup melted butter

    o   Pinch of salt

- **For the Filling:**

    o   4 oz cream cheese, softened

    o   3 oz full-fat ricotta cheese

    o   1/4 cup granulated sugar substitute (suitable for baking)

    o   2 large eggs

    o   1 teaspoon vanilla extract

    o   Lemon zest (optional)

Preparation:

1. Preheat oven to 325°F (163°C).

2. **Make the Crust:** Combine almond flour, melted butter, and salt in a bowl. Press the mixture into the bottom of a springform pan. Bake for 10 minutes, then let cool slightly.

3. **Make the Filling:** In a large bowl, beat together cream cheese and ricotta cheese until smooth.

4. Add the sugar substitute, eggs one at a time, vanilla extract, and lemon zest (if using). Beat until well combined.

5. Pour the filling over the cooled crust.

6. Bake for 50-60 minutes, or until the center is slightly set but still jiggles slightly.

7. Turn off the oven and let the cheesecake cool completely in the oven with the door cracked open.

8. Refrigerate for at least 4 hours, or ideally overnight, before serving.

Nutritional Value (per serving):

- Calories: 450

- Fat: 35g

- Protein: 8g

- Net Carbs: 5g (depending on the sugar substitute used)

2. Almond Flour Brownies

Ingredients:

- 1 cup almond flour

- 1/4 cup unsweetened cocoa powder

- 1/4 teaspoon baking powder

- 1/4 teaspoon salt

- 1/2 cup butter, softened

- 3 large eggs

- 1/2 cup granulated sugar substitute (suitable for baking)

- 1 teaspoon vanilla extract

- 1/2 cup chopped nuts (optional)

Preparation:

1. Preheat oven to 350°F (175°C).

2. Grease an 8x8 inch baking pan.

3. In a medium bowl, whisk together almond flour, cocoa powder, baking powder, and salt.

4. In a separate bowl, cream together softened butter and sugar substitute until light and fluffy. Beat in eggs one at a time, then stir in vanilla extract.

5. Gradually add the dry ingredients to the wet ingredients, mixing until just combined. Fold in chopped nuts (if using).

6. Pour the batter into the prepared baking pan.

7. Bake for 20-25 minutes, or until a toothpick inserted into the center comes out with a few moist crumbs.

8. Let the brownies cool completely in the pan before cutting into squares.

Nutritional Value (per serving):

- Calories: 350

- Fat: 25g

- Protein: 6g

- Net Carbs: 5g (depending on the sugar substitute used)

3. Coconut Macaroons

Ingredients:

- 2 cups unsweetened shredded coconut

- 3 large egg whites

- 1/4 cup granulated sugar substitute (suitable for baking)

- Pinch of salt

Preparation:

1. Preheat oven to 350°F (175°C).

2. Line a baking sheet with parchment paper.

3. In a large bowl, whisk together egg whites and sugar substitute until stiff peaks form.

4. Gently fold in the shredded coconut until evenly distributed.

5. Using a spoon or cookie scoop, drop heaping tablespoons of the mixture onto the prepared baking sheet.

6. Bake for 15-20 minutes, or until golden brown.

7. Let the macaroons cool completely on the baking sheet before storing in an airtight container.

Nutritional Value (per serving):

- Calories: 150

- Fat: 12g

- Protein: 2g

Chapter 26:
Beverages

1. Green Protein Smoothie:

- Blend: 1 cup unsweetened almond milk, 1 scoop protein powder (unflavored or vanilla), 1 handful spinach, 1/2 avocado, 1/4 cup frozen berries.

2. Chocolate Dream Shake:

- Blend: 1 cup unsweetened coconut milk, 1 scoop chocolate protein powder, 1 tablespoon cocoa powder, 1/4 cup chopped zucchini, 1 tablespoon almond butter, ice cubes (optional).

3. Berry Blast:

- Blend: 1 cup water, 1/2 cup frozen mixed berries, 1/4 cup plain Greek yogurt, 1 tablespoon chia seeds, stevia to taste.

Tips:

- Use low-carb vegetables like spinach, zucchini, or kale to add volume and nutrients.

- Choose unsweetened nut milks like almond milk or coconut milk for a low-carb base.

- Sweeten with natural options like stevia, erythritol, or a small amount of berries.

- Add healthy fats like avocado, nut butter, or chia seeds for satiety.

Flavorful and Hydrating: Infused Water Recipes

1. Citrus Splash:

- Add slices of lemon, lime, orange, or grapefruit to a pitcher of water.

- Let it infuse for at least 30 minutes or overnight for a stronger flavor.

- Experiment with combinations like cucumber-lime or strawberry-mint.

2. Berry Bliss:

- Add a handful of raspberries, blueberries, or blackberries to a pitcher of water.

- Consider muddling the berries slightly to release more flavor.

- You can add a sprig of mint or rosemary for an extra touch.

3. Ginger Kick:

- Add a few slices of fresh ginger to a pitcher of water.

- For a spicier drink, consider adding a thin slice of jalapeno (remove seeds for less heat).

- Let it infuse for at least 30 minutes for a refreshing and invigorating drink.

Creamy and Keto-Friendly Coffee Drinks:

1. Bulletproof Coffee:

- Blend: 1 cup brewed coffee, 1 tablespoon grass-fed butter or MCT oil, a pinch of cinnamon.

- This creates a rich and creamy coffee with added healthy fats.

2. Keto Vanilla Latte:

- Froth 1 cup unsweetened almond milk or coconut milk.

- Combine brewed coffee with the frothed milk, 1 teaspoon vanilla extract, and a few drops of stevia (optional).

3. Spiced Mocha:

- Combine brewed coffee with unsweetened almond milk, 1/2 teaspoon unsweetened cocoa powder, a pinch of cinnamon, and a pinch of ground nutmeg.

- Sweeten with a few drops of stevia (optional).

Tips:

- Use unsweetened nut milks or heavy cream for a richer and creamier coffee.

- Sweeten with keto-friendly options like stevia, erythritol, or a small amount of unsweetened cocoa powder.

- Experiment with different spices like cinnamon, nutmeg, or cardamom for added flavor variations.

Chapter 27:

Holiday and Special Occasion Recipes

A Festive Keto Feast: Thanksgiving to Birthday

Thanksgiving:

- **Keto-Friendly Turkey**: Roast a whole turkey using your preferred method. Season generously with herbs and spices like rosemary, thyme, sage, and pepper. Consider brining the turkey for extra flavor and moisture (use a sugar-free brine recipe).

- **Keto Stuffing:** Ditch the traditional bread-based stuffing and opt for a delicious and flavorful alternative. Here are some options:

  - **Sausage and Cauliflower Stuffing:** Saute chopped sausage with onions and celery.

Add riced cauliflower, chopped nuts, and seasonings like sage, thyme, and rosemary. Bake until golden brown and bubbly.

o **Mushroom and Herb Stuffing**: Saute a variety of mushrooms with onions and garlic. Add chopped fresh herbs like parsley, thyme, and chives. Mix with cooked and crumbled chicken sausage (optional) and bake until fragrant and heated through.

- **Roasted Vegetables:** Roast a variety of low-carb vegetables like Brussels sprouts, broccoli, asparagus, and cauliflower with olive oil, salt, pepper, and your favorite herbs. Consider tossing them with chopped pecans or walnuts for added crunch.

Christmas:

- **Keto Roast Beef:** Slow-roast a well-marbled cut of beef like ribeye or prime rib. Season generously and cook to your desired doneness.

- **Creamy Cauliflower Mash:** A classic mashed potato substitute. Steam or boil riced cauliflower until tender. Mash with cream cheese, butter, and seasonings like garlic powder, chives, and salt.

- **Green Beans with Bacon:** Saute green beans with crispy bacon bits. Add a splash of low-carb broth and seasonings like Dijon mustard and black pepper for a flavorful side dish.

Keto-Friendly Birthday Cake:

Here are two options to satisfy your sweet tooth on your birthday:

- **Almond Flour Cake:** This cake uses almond flour, eggs, and a sugar substitute to create a moist and delicious base. You can frost it with a keto-friendly cream cheese frosting or whipped cream sweetened with stevia or erythritol.

- **Cheesecake Bars:** Individual cheesecake bars are another great option. Use a keto-friendly crust made with almond flour and butter, and a filling with cream cheese, eggs, and a sugar substitute. Top with fresh berries for a festive touch.

Tips:

- Research and choose keto-friendly recipes for your specific dishes. Many recipe websites offer low-carb variations of classic holiday favorites.

- Get creative with substitutions. Use cauliflower rice for dishes that traditionally call for grains.

- Focus on whole, unprocessed ingredients for a healthy and delicious keto feast.

- Don't forget to adjust portion sizes based on your individual needs.

CONCLUSION

In closing, embracing a ketogenic diet doesn't have to mean sacrificing taste or festivity. From satisfying snacks to decadent desserts, there's a world of delicious choices waiting to be explored. With a little creativity and these recipe ideas as inspiration, you can craft keto-friendly meals that cater to any event, from a cozy weeknight dinner to a show-stopping holiday feast.

Remember, the key to success lies in focusing on whole, unprocessed foods and finding substitutions that suit your taste preferences. Don't be afraid to explore! There are countless low-carb alternatives for classic dishes, and with a little study, you can discover hidden gems in the keto recipe world.

This journey isn't just about restriction; it's about accepting a new way of appreciating food. By exploring the unique flavors and textures offered by low-carb ingredients, you can build a vibrant and satisfying relationship with food that fuels your body and delights your taste buds.

Here are some final thoughts to keep in mind as you start on your keto culinary adventure:

Prioritize Planning: A little meal planning goes a long way, especially when starting a new diet. Research recipes, make grocery lists, and prep ingredients in advance to avoid unhealthy temptations.

Embrace Variety: Don't get stuck in a rut! Explore different cuisines and play with new low-carb ingredients. There's a whole world of flavor waiting to be found beyond the standard keto fare.

Find Your Tribe: Surround yourself with others who understand your food choices. Online forums, social media groups, and even local keto meetups can provide useful support and inspiration.

Listen to Your Body: Pay attention to how your body responds to different foods. Adjust your approach as needed, and don't be afraid to consult a healthcare professional or registered dietitian for personalized advice.

Ultimately, a good keto journey is about creating a sustainable and enjoyable lifestyle. By incorporating these tips and the recipe ideas offered, you can start on a delicious and rewarding exploration of the ketogenic world. So, fire up your oven, unleash your creativity, and get ready to experience a whole new level of healthy and satisfying cuisine

THANKS

READER